I0701413

Fatty Liver Diet Cookbook

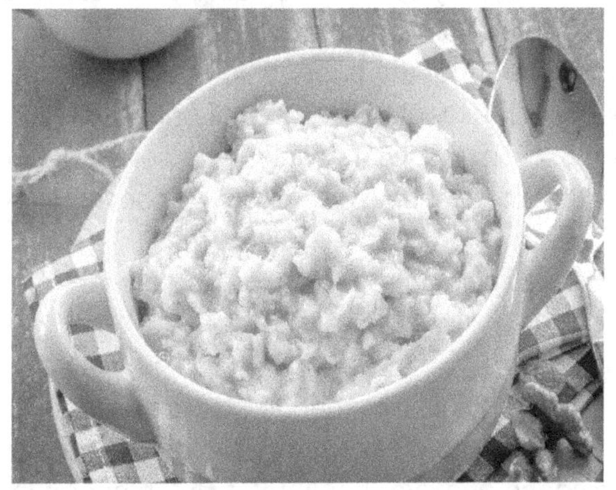

Nourishing Recipes to Fuel Your Day
and Support Liver Wellness

Isaac Hendricks

Copyright © 2024 [ISAAC HENDRICKS]

All rights reserved. No part of this publication may be reproduced, distributed, or transmitted in any form or by any means, including photocopying, recording, or other electronic or mechanical methods, without the prior written permission of the publisher, except in the case of brief quotations embodied in critical reviews and certain other noncommercial uses permitted by copyright law.

For permission requests, please contact the publisher.

This book is intended to provide general information and guidance on the topic of fatty liver disease and liver health. It is not intended to replace professional medical advice, diagnosis, or treatment. Readers are encouraged to consult with a qualified healthcare professional regarding any medical concerns or questions they may have. The author and publisher disclaim any liability arising directly or indirectly from the use of this book.

Table of Contents

INTRODUCTION

Welcome to the "Fatty Liver Diet Cookbook," a comprehensive guide to managing and improving fatty liver disease through nutrition and lifestyle changes. Fatty liver disease, also known as hepatic steatosis, is a condition characterised by the accumulation of fat in the liver cells. It can be caused by various factors, including obesity, insulin resistance, high alcohol consumption, and certain medications.

In recent years, the prevalence of fatty liver disease has been on the rise, largely due to the increasing rates of obesity and metabolic syndrome. Left untreated, fatty liver disease can progress to more severe conditions such as non-alcoholic steatohepatitis (NASH), liver fibrosis, cirrhosis, and even liver cancer. However, the good news is that fatty liver disease is often reversible, especially in its early stages, through lifestyle modifications such as diet and exercise.

This book aims to provide you with the knowledge, tools, and delicious recipes necessary to support your liver health and manage fatty liver disease effectively. Each chapter will delve into different aspects of the condition, from understanding its causes and symptoms to implementing a personalised diet plan tailored to your needs. You'll discover the importance of essential nutrients for liver health, learn how to create balanced and nutritious meals, and explore a variety of flavorful recipes designed to nourish your body and support optimal liver function.

Whether you've recently been diagnosed with fatty liver disease or are looking to improve your liver health preventatively, this book is your ultimate guide to reclaiming control of your health and vitality.
By adopting a wholesome and liver-friendly diet, you can take proactive steps towards reversing liver damage, reducing inflammation, and restoring your overall well-being. Let's embark on this journey together towards a healthier, happier you!

Brief Explanation:
Understanding Fatty Liver: Causes and Symptoms
Fatty liver disease is a condition characterised by the accumulation of fat in the liver cells. While it's normal to have some fat in the liver, when more than 5-10% of the liver's weight is fat, it's considered fatty liver disease. There are two main types of fatty liver disease:

alcoholic fatty liver disease and non-alcoholic fatty liver disease (NAFLD).
Alcoholic fatty liver disease is caused by excessive alcohol consumption, which can lead to fat accumulation in the liver and inflammation. On the other hand, NAFLD is not related to alcohol consumption and is commonly associated with

obesity, insulin resistance, type 2 diabetes, high cholesterol, and metabolic syndrome.
Symptoms of fatty liver disease can vary depending on the severity of the condition.

In the early stages, many people may not experience any noticeable symptoms, while others may experience fatigue, weakness, abdominal discomfort, and an enlarged liver. As the disease progresses, it can lead to more serious complications such as liver fibrosis, cirrhosis, and liver cancer.

Risk factors for fatty liver disease include obesity, insulin resistance, type 2 diabetes, high cholesterol, metabolic syndrome, and excessive alcohol consumption. Certain medications, genetic factors, and rapid weight loss can also increase the risk of developing fatty liver disease.

Diagnosing fatty liver disease typically involves a combination of medical history, physical examination, blood tests, imaging studies (such as ultrasound, CT scan, or MRI), and sometimes a liver biopsy. Early detection and intervention are crucial for preventing the progression of fatty liver disease and reducing the risk of complications.

In Chapter 1, we will go deeper into the causes, risk factors, and symptoms of fatty liver disease, providing you with a solid understanding of this condition and its implications for your health. We'll also discuss the importance of early detection and proactive management strategies to support liver health and overall well-being. Get ready to empower yourself with knowledge and take control of your liver health journey!

CHAPTER ONE

Understanding Fatty Liver

Causes and Symptoms

Fatty liver disease, a condition characterised by the accumulation of fat in the liver cells, has become increasingly prevalent in recent years, posing a significant public health concern worldwide. This chapter aims to provide a comprehensive overview of the causes, risk factors, and symptoms of fatty liver disease, shedding light on this complex condition and its implications for overall health and well-being.

Causes of Fatty Liver Disease:
There are two primary types of fatty liver disease: alcoholic fatty liver disease (AFLD) and non-alcoholic fatty liver disease (NAFLD). While both conditions involve the accumulation of fat in the liver, they differ in their underlying causes.

Alcoholic Fatty Liver Disease (AFLD):
As the name suggests, alcoholic fatty liver disease is directly linked to excessive alcohol consumption. When alcohol is consumed, it is metabolised by the liver, where it undergoes chemical reactions that can lead to the production of harmful substances and oxidative stress. Over time, chronic alcohol abuse can overwhelm the liver's ability to process

fat, resulting in the accumulation of fat droplets within the liver cells.

The severity of AFLD can vary depending on factors such as the amount and duration of alcohol consumption, genetic predisposition, and overall health status. In its early stages, AFLD may manifest as fatty liver, a reversible condition that can improve with abstinence from alcohol. However, continued alcohol abuse can progress to more severe forms of liver disease, including alcoholic hepatitis, liver fibrosis, cirrhosis, and even liver failure.

Non-Alcoholic Fatty Liver Disease (NAFLD):
Unlike AFLD, NAFLD is not related to alcohol consumption and is instead associated with metabolic factors such as obesity, insulin resistance, type 2 diabetes, high cholesterol, and metabolic syndrome. The exact mechanisms underlying NAFLD are complex and multifactorial, involving a combination of genetic, environmental, and lifestyle factors.

In NAFLD, the accumulation of fat in the liver is primarily driven by insulin resistance, which impairs the liver's ability to regulate glucose and lipid metabolism effectively. As a result, excess fat from the bloodstream is deposited in the liver, leading to the development of fatty liver disease. Other contributing factors to NAFLD include dietary habits, sedentary lifestyle, hormonal imbalances, and gut microbiota dysbiosis.

Risk Factors for Fatty Liver Disease

Several factors can increase the risk of developing fatty liver disease, regardless of whether it is alcoholic or non-alcoholic in nature. Understanding these risk factors is crucial for early detection and proactive management of the condition. Some of the key risk factors include:

1. **Obesity:** Excess body weight, particularly visceral adiposity, is strongly associated with an increased risk of fatty liver disease. Obesity contributes to insulin resistance, inflammation, and dyslipidemia, all of which can promote the accumulation of fat in the liver.

2. **Insulin Resistance and Type 2 Diabetes:** Insulin resistance, a hallmark of metabolic syndrome and type 2 diabetes, plays a central role in the pathogenesis of NAFLD. Insulin resistance impairs the liver's ability to respond to insulin, leading to dysregulated glucose and lipid metabolism, which can predispose to fatty liver disease.

3. **High Cholesterol and Triglycerides:** Elevated levels of cholesterol and triglycerides in the bloodstream can

promote the accumulation of fat in the liver and contribute to the development of NAFLD. Dyslipidemia is commonly observed in individuals with metabolic syndrome and insulin resistance, further exacerbating liver fat accumulation.

4. **Metabolic Syndrome:** Metabolic syndrome is a cluster of metabolic abnormalities, including central obesity, insulin resistance, dyslipidemia, and hypertension. Individuals with metabolic syndrome are at significantly higher risk of developing NAFLD and its associated complications.

5. **Excessive Alcohol Consumption:** Chronic and excessive alcohol consumption is a major risk factor for alcoholic fatty liver disease. The toxic effects of alcohol on the liver can disrupt lipid metabolism, promote inflammation, and lead to the accumulation of fat in the liver cells.

6. **Medications and Toxins:** Certain medications, such as corticosteroids, tamoxifen, methotrexate, and antiretroviral drugs, can increase the risk of developing fatty liver disease by impairing liver function or promoting fat accumulation. Exposure to environmental toxins, industrial chemicals, and pesticides may also contribute to liver damage and fatty liver disease.

Symptoms of Fatty Liver Disease

In its early stages, fatty liver disease may not cause any noticeable symptoms, making it challenging to diagnose without medical evaluation. However, as the condition progresses, various symptoms and complications may arise, reflecting the extent of liver damage and dysfunction. Common symptoms of fatty liver disease include:

1. **Fatigue and Weakness:** Many individuals with fatty liver disease experience persistent fatigue and weakness, which can significantly impact daily functioning and quality of life. Fatigue is often attributed to liver inflammation, impaired energy metabolism, and systemic effects of chronic inflammation.

2. **Abdominal Discomfort:** Some people with fatty liver disease may experience mild to moderate discomfort or pain in the upper right abdomen, where the liver is located. This discomfort may be dull, achy, or tender and is often exacerbated by fatty or greasy foods.

3. **Enlarged Liver:** In some cases, fatty liver disease can cause the liver to become enlarged, a condition known as hepatomegaly. Enlargement of the liver may be detected during a physical examination

or imaging studies and is indicative of liver inflammation and fat accumulation.

4. **Elevated Liver Enzymes:** Blood tests may reveal elevated levels of liver enzymes, such as alanine transaminase (ALT) and aspartate transaminase (AST), indicating liver inflammation and damage. However, it's important to note that not all individuals with fatty liver disease will have abnormal liver enzyme levels, especially in the early stages of the condition.

5. **Complications:** As fatty liver disease progresses, it can lead to more serious complications such as liver fibrosis, cirrhosis, and hepatocellular carcinoma (liver cancer). These complications may manifest with symptoms such as jaundice (yellowing of the skin and eyes), abdominal swelling (ascites), easy bruising or bleeding, and confusion (hepatic encephalopathy).

Diagnosing Fatty Liver Disease

Diagnosing fatty liver disease typically involves a combination of medical history, physical examination, laboratory tests, imaging studies, and sometimes a liver biopsy. During a medical history review, your healthcare provider will inquire about your symptoms, medical history, alcohol consumption, medications, and risk factors for liver disease. A physical examination may reveal signs of liver enlargement, tenderness, or other abdominal abnormalities.

Blood tests are commonly used to assess liver function and detect abnormalities in liver enzymes, such as ALT, AST, alkaline phosphatase (ALP), gamma-glutamyl transferase (GGT), and bilirubin. Elevated levels of these enzymes may indicate liver inflammation, damage, or impaired liver function. Additionally, blood tests may be used to evaluate other parameters such as cholesterol, triglycerides, glucose, insulin, and markers of inflammation.

Imaging studies such as ultrasound, computed tomography (CT) scan, or magnetic resonance imaging (MRI) may be performed to visualise the liver and assess for the presence of fat, inflammation, or other structural abnormalities. Ultrasound is often the initial imaging modality of choice for diagnosing fatty liver disease due to its widespread availability, cost-effectiveness,

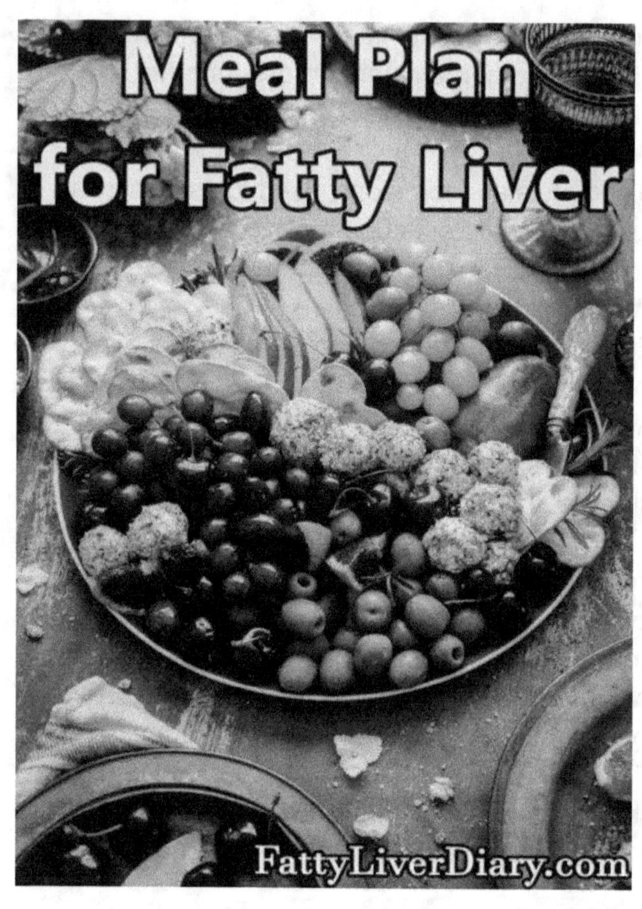

Meal Plan
for Fatty Liver
FattyLiverDiary.com

CHAPTER TWO

The Role of Diet in Managing Fatty Liver Disease

Diet plays a crucial role in the management and prevention of fatty liver disease. In this chapter, we will explore the impact of dietary choices on liver health, discuss key nutrients and foods that support liver function, and provide practical strategies for crafting a nutritious and liver-friendly diet plan.

Importance of Diet in Fatty Liver Disease Management:
1. The liver is a central organ involved in the metabolism of nutrients, toxins, and waste products, making it highly susceptible to the effects of dietary intake. A diet high in unhealthy fats, sugars, and processed foods can contribute to liver inflammation, oxidative stress, and fat accumulation, exacerbating fatty liver disease.

Conversely, adopting a balanced and nutrient-rich diet can help alleviate liver damage, reduce inflammation, and support optimal liver function. Dietary modifications, along with lifestyle changes such as regular exercise and weight management, are cornerstone interventions in the management of fatty liver disease.

Key Nutrients for Liver Health:

2. Several nutrients have been shown to play a crucial role in promoting liver health and mitigating the progression of fatty liver disease. These include:

- **Omega-3 Fatty Acids:** Found in fatty fish (such as salmon, mackerel, and sardines), flaxseeds, chia seeds, and walnuts, omega-3 fatty acids have anti-inflammatory properties and may help reduce liver fat accumulation and inflammation.

- **Antioxidants:** Antioxidant-rich foods such as fruits (berries, citrus fruits), vegetables (leafy greens, cruciferous vegetables), and herbs/spices (turmeric, garlic, ginger) help combat oxidative stress and protect liver cells from damage.

- **Fibre:** Soluble fibre, found in foods like oats, legumes, fruits, and vegetables, helps regulate blood sugar levels, promote satiety, and support healthy gut microbiota, all of which are beneficial for liver health.

- **Vitamin E:** Vitamin E, found in nuts, seeds, vegetable oils, and leafy greens, is a potent antioxidant that may help reduce liver inflammation and oxidative stress in individuals with fatty liver disease.

- **Choline:** Choline, found in eggs, lean meats, poultry, fish, and cruciferous vegetables, is essential for liver function, fat metabolism, and the production of phosphatidylcholine, a component of cell membranes.

Foods to Include in a Fatty Liver Diet:

3. When crafting a diet plan for fatty liver disease, it's important to focus on whole, nutrient-dense foods that support liver health and overall well-being. Some examples of foods to include in a fatty liver diet include:

- **Lean Protein Sources:** Incorporate lean protein sources such as poultry, fish, tofu, legumes, and low-fat dairy products into your meals to support muscle maintenance and repair without contributing to excess fat intake.

- **Colourful Fruits and Vegetables:** Aim to include a variety of colourful fruits and vegetables in your diet, as they are rich in vitamins, minerals, antioxidants, and phytonutrients that support liver detoxification and reduce inflammation.

- **Whole Grains:** Choose whole grains such as oats, quinoa, brown rice, barley, and whole wheat bread over refined grains to increase fibre intake, stabilise blood sugar levels, and promote satiety.

- **Healthy Fats:** Opt for healthy fats such as avocado, olive oil, nuts, seeds, and fatty fish, which provide essential fatty acids and have anti-inflammatory properties that benefit liver health.

- **Dairy Alternatives:** If you have lactose intolerance or prefer dairy-free options, consider incorporating fortified plant-based milk alternatives such as almond milk, soy milk, or oat milk into your diet for calcium and vitamin D.

Foods to Limit or Avoid:

4. In addition to emphasising nutrient-rich foods, it's important to minimise or avoid certain dietary components that can exacerbate fatty liver disease and promote liver damage. These include:

- **Saturated and Trans Fats:** Limit consumption of saturated fats found in red meat, processed meats, full-fat dairy products, and fried foods, as well as trans fats found in partially hydrogenated oils and processed foods.

- **Added Sugars and Refined Carbohydrates:** Reduce intake of added sugars from sugary beverages, sweets, pastries, and processed foods, as well as refined carbohydrates such as white bread, white rice, and sugary cereals, which can contribute to insulin resistance and liver fat accumulation.

- **Excessive Alcohol:** If you have alcoholic fatty liver disease or are at risk of developing liver disease, it's essential to avoid or limit alcohol consumption to prevent further liver damage and promote recovery.

Practical Tips for Implementing a Fatty Liver Diet:

5. Transitioning to a fatty liver diet can be challenging, but with the right strategies and mindset, it's entirely achievable. Here are some practical tips for incorporating liver-friendly eating habits into your daily routine:

- **Plan and Prepare Meals:** Take time to plan and prepare nutritious meals and snacks ahead of time to avoid relying on convenience foods or unhealthy options when hunger strikes.

- **Read Food Labels:** Learn to read food labels and ingredient lists to identify hidden sources of added sugars, unhealthy fats, and artificial additives in packaged foods.

- **Practice Portion Control:** Be mindful of portion sizes and aim to balance your plate with a variety of nutrient-dense foods, including lean proteins, colourful vegetables, whole grains, and healthy fats.

- **Stay Hydrated:** Drink plenty of water throughout the day to stay hydrated and support optimal liver function. Limit intake of sugary beverages and opt for water, herbal tea, or infused water instead.

- **Seek Support:** Don't hesitate to seek support from healthcare professionals, registered dietitians, or support groups specialising in liver health and nutrition. They can provide personalised guidance, resources, and encouragement to help you achieve your dietary goals.

In summary, diet plays a pivotal role in the management and prevention of fatty liver disease. By adopting a balanced and liver-friendly diet rich in essential nutrients and whole foods while minimising intake of unhealthy fats, sugars, and alcohol, you can support liver health, reduce inflammation, and improve overall well-being.

Remember, small changes in dietary habits can yield significant benefits for liver health over time. Stay committed to making positive choices and nourishing your body with the fuel it needs to thrive.

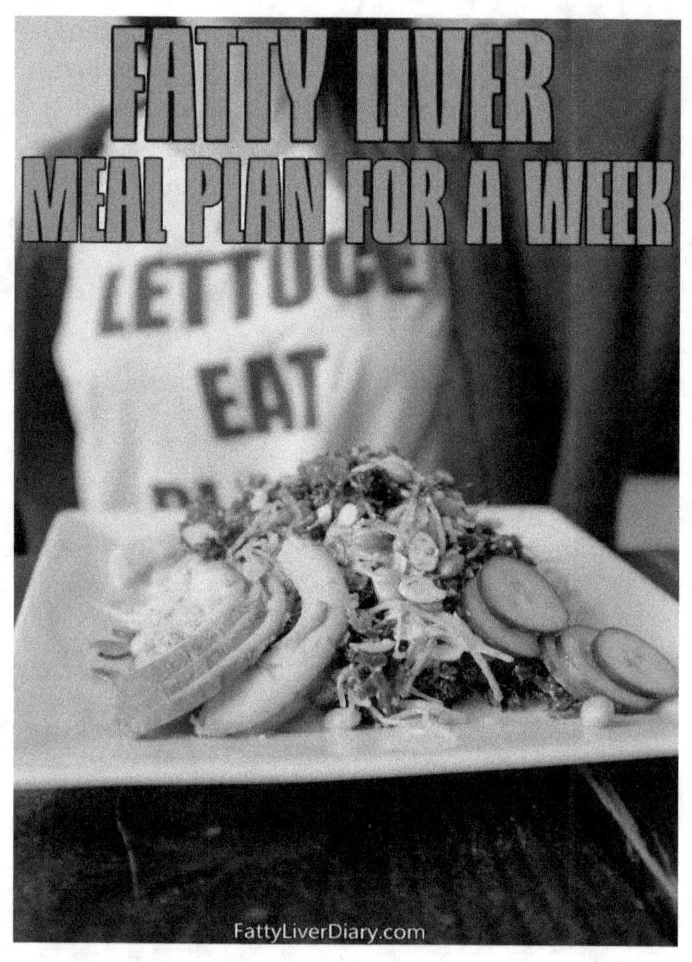

FATTY LIVER
MEAL PLAN FOR A WEEK
LETTUCE
EAT
FattyLiverDiary.com

CHAPTER THREE

Essential Nutrients for a Healthy Liver

Welcome to Chapter 3 of the "Fatty Liver Diet Cookbook," where we explore the essential nutrients your liver needs to thrive. In this chapter, we will dive into the vital vitamins, minerals, and other nutrients that play a crucial role in supporting liver health and managing fatty liver disease. By understanding the importance of these nutrients and incorporating them into your diet, you can nourish your liver and promote optimal function.

Vitamins for Liver Health:

1. **Vitamin E:** This powerful antioxidant helps protect liver cells from damage caused by oxidative stress and inflammation. Sources of vitamin E include nuts, seeds, leafy greens, and vegetable oils.

2. **Vitamin C:** Another potent antioxidant, vitamin C supports liver detoxification processes and helps boost the immune system. Citrus fruits, strawberries, bell peppers, and broccoli are excellent sources of vitamin C.

3. **Vitamin D:** Adequate vitamin D levels are essential for liver health, as this vitamin plays a role in reducing liver inflammation and improving insulin sensitivity. Sunlight exposure, fatty fish, fortified dairy products, and egg yolks are sources of vitamin D.

4. **Vitamin B Complex:** B vitamins, including B12, B6, and folate, are crucial for energy metabolism, liver detoxification, and the synthesis of liver-supportive compounds. Whole grains, lean meats, eggs, leafy greens, and legumes are rich in B vitamins.

Minerals for Liver Function:

1. **Zinc:** This essential mineral plays a role in liver detoxification processes and helps protect liver cells from damage. Seafood, lean meats, nuts, seeds, and whole grains are good sources of zinc.

2. **Selenium:** Selenium is an antioxidant mineral that supports liver health by reducing oxidative stress and inflammation. Brazil nuts, seafood, poultry, and whole grains are sources of selenium.

3. **Magnesium:** Magnesium plays a role in over 300 enzymatic reactions in the body, including those involved in liver function and detoxification. Leafy greens, nuts, seeds,

whole grains, and legumes are excellent sources of magnesium.

1. **Omega-3 Fatty Acids:** These healthy fats help reduce liver inflammation, improve liver function, and decrease liver fat accumulation. Fatty fish like salmon, mackerel, and sardines, as well as flaxseeds, chia seeds, and walnuts, are rich sources of omega-3 fatty acids.

2. **Antioxidants:** In addition to vitamins E and C, other antioxidants such as glutathione, beta-carotene, and flavonoids help protect liver cells from damage and promote liver detoxification. Colourful fruits and vegetables, herbs, spices, and green tea are abundant sources of antioxidants.

3. **Phytonutrients:** Plant compounds like flavonoids, polyphenols, and carotenoids have anti-inflammatory and hepatoprotective properties that benefit liver health. Including a variety of fruits, vegetables, herbs, and spices in your diet ensures you receive a wide range of phytonutrients.

Summary:

Ensuring adequate intake of essential nutrients is crucial for supporting liver health and managing fatty liver disease. By incorporating a diverse array of vitamins, minerals, antioxidants, and phytonutrients into your diet through whole, nutrient-rich foods, you can provide your liver with the tools it needs to function optimally. Remember to focus on a balanced diet that includes a variety of colourful fruits and vegetables, lean proteins, healthy fats, and whole grains to nourish your liver and promote overall well-being.

CHAPTER FOUR

Crafting Your Fatty Liver Diet Plan

In Chapter 4 of the "Fatty Liver Diet Cookbook," We will guide you through the process of crafting a personalised diet plan to support your liver health and manage fatty liver disease effectively. In this chapter, we'll explore step-by-step strategies for designing a nutritious and sustainable eating plan that suits your preferences, lifestyle, and nutritional needs.

Understanding Your Dietary Goals

Before diving into crafting your fatty liver diet plan, it's essential to clarify your dietary goals and objectives. Whether your primary focus is reducing liver fat, improving liver function, managing weight, or enhancing overall health, defining your goals will help tailor your diet plan to meet your specific needs and preferences.

Step 1: Assess Your Current Eating Habits
Take some time to reflect on your current eating habits, preferences, and dietary patterns. Consider the types of foods you typically consume, portion sizes, meal timing, snacking habits, and any challenges or obstacles you may encounter when trying to make dietary changes.

Step 2: Identify Areas for Improvement
Next, identify areas of your diet that may need improvement to support liver health and manage fatty liver disease. This may include reducing intake of high-sugar and high-fat foods, increasing consumption of fruits and vegetables, incorporating more lean proteins and whole grains, and practising portion control.

Step 3: Set Realistic and Achievable Goals
Based on your dietary assessment, set realistic and achievable goals that align with your overarching objectives. Break down your goals into smaller, manageable steps to make them more attainable and sustainable over the long term. Whether it's swapping out sugary beverages for water, adding an extra serving of vegetables to your meals, or cooking more homemade meals, start with small changes and gradually build momentum.

Step 4: Design Your Fatty Liver Diet Plan
Now it's time to design your personalised fatty liver diet plan.
Consider the following components when crafting your plan:

1. **Macronutrient Distribution:** Aim for a balanced distribution of macronutrients, including carbohydrates, proteins, and fats, to support overall health and liver function. While there's no one-size-fits-all approach, a general guideline is to prioritise complex

carbohydrates, lean proteins, and healthy fats while limiting added sugars and saturated fats.

2. **Portion Control:** Practice portion control to manage calorie intake and prevent overeating, which can contribute to weight gain and liver fat accumulation. Use visual cues, portion control tools, and mindful eating practices to gauge appropriate portion sizes and prevent excessive calorie consumption.

3. **Meal Timing:** Establish a regular eating schedule with meals and snacks spaced evenly throughout the day to maintain stable blood sugar levels and prevent energy dips. Aim to eat every 3-4 hours to keep hunger at bay and provide your body with a steady source of nutrients.

4. **Food Choices:** Choose nutrient-dense, whole foods that nourish your body and support liver health. Emphasise fruits, vegetables, whole grains, lean proteins, healthy fats, and plant-based sources of protein and fibre. Minimise intake of processed foods, sugary snacks, fried foods, high-fat dairy products.

5. **Hydration:** Stay hydrated by drinking plenty of water throughout the day to support liver function, aid digestion, and promote overall health. Aim for at least 8-10 cups of water daily, and adjust your fluid intake based on factors such as activity level, climate, and individual hydration needs.

6. **Variety and Balance:** Incorporate a variety of foods from all food groups into your diet to ensure you receive a wide range of nutrients and phytonutrients. Aim for a colourful plate with plenty of fruits and vegetables, lean proteins, whole grains, and healthy fats to maximise nutrient intake and promote dietary diversity.

Step 5: Implement and Monitor Your Plan
Once you've crafted your fatty liver diet plan, it's time to put it into action and monitor your progress. Stay consistent with your dietary changes, track your food intake, and pay attention to how your body responds to different foods and eating patterns. Be flexible and willing to adjust your plan as needed based on your evolving goals, preferences, and feedback from your body.

Summary:

Crafting a personalised fatty liver diet plan is an essential step towards supporting liver health, managing fatty liver disease, and promoting overall well-being. By assessing your current eating habits, setting realistic goals, designing a balanced and nutritious meal plan, and implementing mindful eating practices, you can empower yourself to take control of your health and make positive dietary changes that support your liver for years to come. Remember, small changes can lead to significant improvements over time, so start where you are and take consistent steps towards a healthier lifestyle.

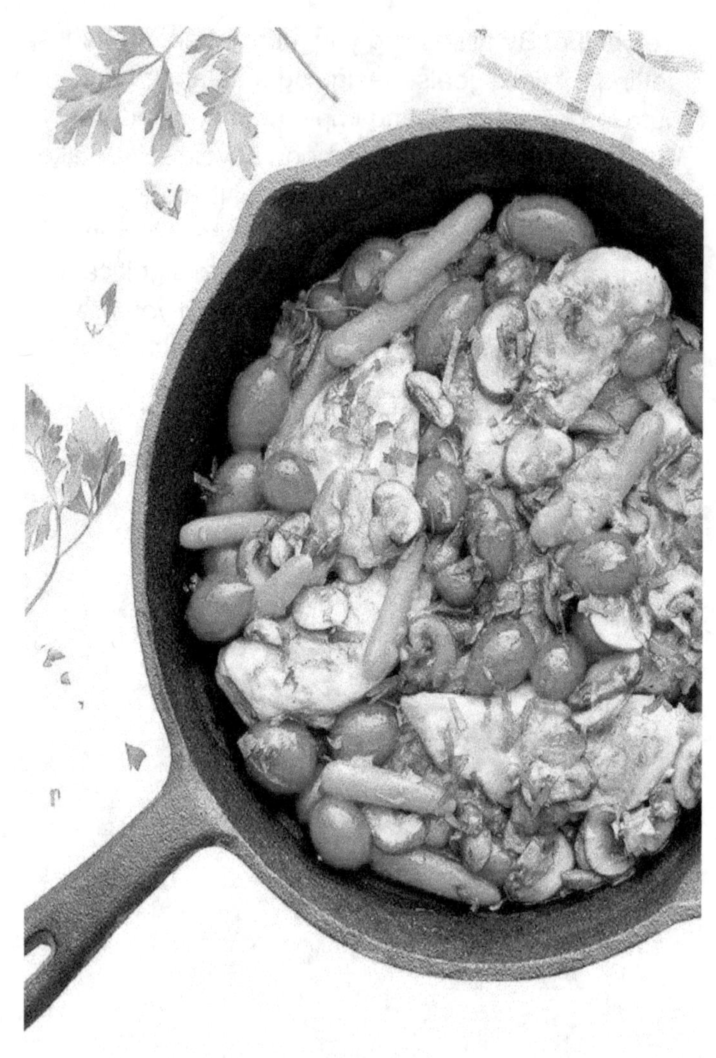

CHAPTER FIVE

Delicious and Nutritious Breakfast Recipes

In this Chapter of the "Fatty Liver Diet Cookbook," we are discussing the most important meal of the day; breakfast.

We will explore a collection of delicious and nutritious breakfast recipes designed to nourish your body, support liver health, and kick-start your day with energy and vitality. From hearty oatmeal creations to satisfying egg dishes and refreshing smoothie bowls, these recipes are as flavorful as they are beneficial for your well-being.

1. Hearty Quinoa Breakfast Bowl:
    - **Ingredients:**
        1. 1/2 cup cooked quinoa
        2. 1/4 cup Greek yoghourt
        3. 1 tablespoon honey or maple syrup
        4. 1/4 cup mixed berries (strawberries, blueberries, raspberries)
        5. 1 tablespoon chopped nuts or seeds (walnuts, almonds, chia seeds)

- **Instructions:**
    1. In a bowl, combine the cooked quinoa, Greek yoghurt, and honey or maple syrup.
    2. Top with mixed berries and chopped nuts or seeds for added flavour, texture, and nutrients.
    3. Stir gently to combine, then dig in and enjoy this satisfying and protein-packed breakfast option.

2. Vegetable Egg Muffins:
    - **Ingredients:**
        1. 6 large eggs
        2. 1/4 cup diced bell peppers
        3. 1/4 cup diced tomatoes
        4. 1/4 cup chopped spinach
        5. 1/4 cup diced onions
        6. Salt and pepper to taste

    - **Instructions:**
        1. Preheat your oven to 350°F (175°C) and lightly grease a muffin tin with cooking spray.
        2. In a mixing bowl, beat the eggs until well combined.

3. Stir in the diced bell peppers, tomatoes, spinach, onions, salt, and pepper.
4. Pour the egg mixture evenly into the prepared muffin tin, filling each cup about three-quarters full.
5. Bake in the preheated oven for 20-25 minutes, or until the egg muffins are set and lightly golden on top.
6. Allow the muffins to cool slightly before removing them from the tin.
7. Serve warm or at room temperature for a convenient and protein-rich breakfast on the go.

3. Green Smoothie Power Bowl:
   - **Ingredients:**
     1. 1 cup spinach
     2. 1/2 ripe avocado
     3. 1/2 cup frozen pineapple chunks
     4. 1/2 banana
     5. 1 tablespoon chia seeds
     6. 1/2 cup almond milk
     7. Optional toppings: sliced banana, granola, coconut flakes

- ○ **Instructions:**
    1. In a blender, combine the spinach, avocado, pineapple chunks, banana, chia seeds, and almond milk.
    2. Blend until smooth and creamy, adding more almond milk if needed to reach your desired consistency.
    3. Pour the smoothie into a bowl and top with sliced banana, granola, and coconut flakes for added texture and flavour.
    4. Enjoy this refreshing and nutrient-rich smoothie bowl for a vibrant start to your day.

Conclusion:

These delicious and nutritious breakfast recipes are not only flavorful but also supportive of liver health and overall well-being. Whether you're craving a warm and comforting quinoa breakfast bowl, a protein-packed vegetable egg muffin, or a refreshing green smoothie power bowl, these recipes offer a variety of options to suit your taste preferences and dietary needs. So, fuel your body with the goodness it deserves and enjoy these wholesome breakfast dishes as part of your healthy lifestyle.

CHAPTER SIX

Satisfying Lunch Options for Fatty Liver Health

In this Chapter of the "Fatty Liver Diet Cookbook," readers are treated to a tantalising array of lunch options designed to support liver health and satisfy the palate. Lunchtime presents an opportunity to refuel the body midday with nutritious and flavorful meals that energise and nourish, and this chapter delivers with a diverse selection of recipes that prioritise both taste and wellness.

Before moving into the mouthwatering recipes that await, this chapter opens with an introduction that underscores the importance of lunch in maintaining steady energy levels and supporting overall well-being. Readers are reminded of the significance of choosing balanced, nutrient-dense meals that provide sustained fuel throughout the day while promoting liver health.

Key Principles of Liver-Friendly Lunches

Building upon the foundational knowledge established in earlier chapters, this section outlines the key principles of crafting liver-friendly lunches. Emphasis is placed on incorporating lean proteins, complex carbohydrates, healthy fats, and an abundance of fruits and vegetables into each meal. Readers are encouraged to experiment with a variety of flavours and textures while keeping portion sizes in check to ensure optimal nutrient intake and support liver function.

Recipes for Liver Wellness:
With the groundwork laid, readers are presented with a tantalising array of lunch recipes thoughtfully curated to support liver health and satisfy the senses. From hearty salads and nourishing soups to flavorful sandwiches and wraps, each recipe is designed to be both delicious and nutritious, providing a satisfying midday meal that fuels the body and nourishes the soul.

Sample Recipes:

1. Quinoa Salad with Roasted Vegetables and Herbed Vinaigrette: This vibrant salad features a medley of roasted vegetables, including bell peppers, zucchini, eggplant, and cherry tomatoes, tossed with protein-rich quinoa and a tangy herbed vinaigrette. Packed with fiber, antioxidants, and essential nutrients, this dish is a satisfying lunch option that supports liver health and promotes overall wellness.

2. Turkey and Avocado Wrap with Whole Grain Tortilla: This satisfying wrap combines lean turkey breast, creamy avocado, crisp

lettuce, and sliced tomato wrapped in a whole grain tortilla. Bursting with protein, healthy fats, and fibre, this lunch option provides a balanced combination of nutrients to fuel the body and keep hunger at bay.

3. Lentil and Vegetable Soup: This hearty soup features nutrient-rich lentils simmered with an assortment of vegetables, including carrots, celery, onions, and spinach, in a flavorful broth. Packed with fibre, protein, vitamins, and minerals, this comforting soup is a nourishing lunch option that satisfies the appetite while supporting liver health.

Summary:

As readers reach the conclusion of Chapter 5, they are not just bidding farewell to a collection of recipes—they are embarking on a journey towards wellness, one lunch at a time. With the guidance, inspiration, and delicious recipes found within these pages, they are empowered to make mindful choices that support liver health, nourish their bodies, and delight their taste buds. So, embrace the power of wholesome cuisine, savour the flavours of nutritious meals, and celebrate the joy of nourishing both body and soul.

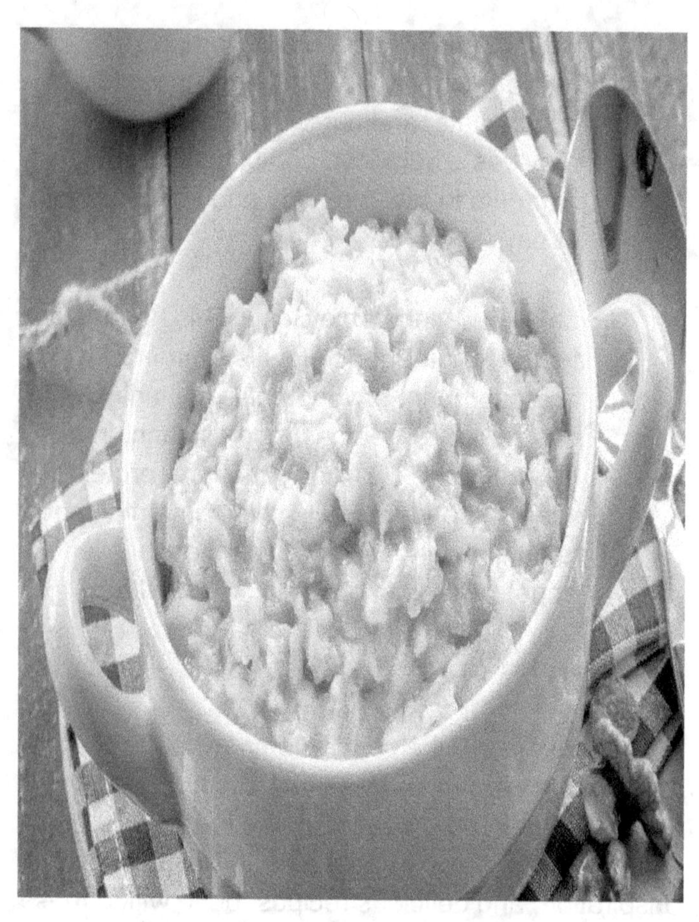

CHAPTER SEVEN

Wholesome Dinner Ideas to Support Liver Function

In Chapter 7 of the "Fatty Liver Diet Cookbook," readers are invited to explore a diverse array of dinner ideas specifically crafted to support liver function and promote overall wellness. As the day winds down and dinner time approaches, this chapter serves as a beacon of inspiration, offering nutritious and delicious meal options that will satisfy both the body and the soul.

Before diving into the tantalising recipes that await, this chapter begins with an introduction that sets the stage for the importance of wholesome dinners in supporting liver health. Readers are reminded of the critical role that dinner plays in the overall dietary landscape and encouraged to approach mealtime with intention, mindfulness, and a commitment to nourishing their bodies from within.

Key Principles of Liver-Friendly Dinners:

Building upon the foundation laid in earlier chapters, this section delves into the key principles of crafting liver-friendly dinners. Readers are reminded of the importance of balance, variety, and moderation in their dietary choices. Emphasis is placed on incorporating nutrient-dense ingredients such as lean proteins, whole grains, and an abundance of colourful fruits and vegetables. Strategies for reducing the intake of processed foods, saturated fats, and added sugars are also highlighted, empowering readers to make informed choices that support liver health.

Recipes for Liver Wellness:

With the groundwork laid, readers are presented with a treasure trove of dinner recipes designed to tantalise the taste buds while nourishing the body. From comforting classics to innovative culinary creations, each recipe is thoughtfully crafted to prioritise flavour, nutrition, and ease of preparation. Whether craving a hearty one-pot meal, a vibrant salad bursting with seasonal produce, or a flavorful vegetarian dish, readers will find options to suit every palate and dietary preference.

Sample Recipes:

1. Grilled Salmon with Lemon-Dill Quinoa: This light and flavorful dish features grilled salmon fillets served atop a bed of fluffy lemon-dill quinoa. Rich in omega-3 fatty acids, protein, and fibre, this dinner option is a powerhouse of nutrients that supports liver health and overall well-being.

2. Mediterranean Chickpea Salad: Bursting with the vibrant flavours of the

Mediterranean, this hearty salad features chickpeas, cherry tomatoes, cucumber, bell peppers, olives, and feta cheese tossed in a zesty lemon-herb dressing. Packed with fibre, antioxidants, and healthy fats, this dish is as satisfying as it is nourishing.

3. Vegetable Stir-Fry with Brown Rice: This quick and easy stir-fry is the perfect way to pack a variety of colourful vegetables into a single meal. Bell peppers, broccoli, carrots, snap peas, and mushrooms are stir-fried to perfection and served over nutty brown rice, creating a deliciously wholesome dinner option that's sure to please the whole family.

Summary:

As readers reach the conclusion of Chapter 6, they are not just bidding farewell to a collection of recipes—they are embarking on a journey towards wellness, one dinner at a time. With the guidance, inspiration, and delicious recipes found within these pages, they are empowered to take control of their health, support their liver function, and nourish their bodies with every meal. So, gather around the dinner table, savour the flavours of wholesome cuisine, and celebrate the power of food to heal, nourish, and rejuvenate.

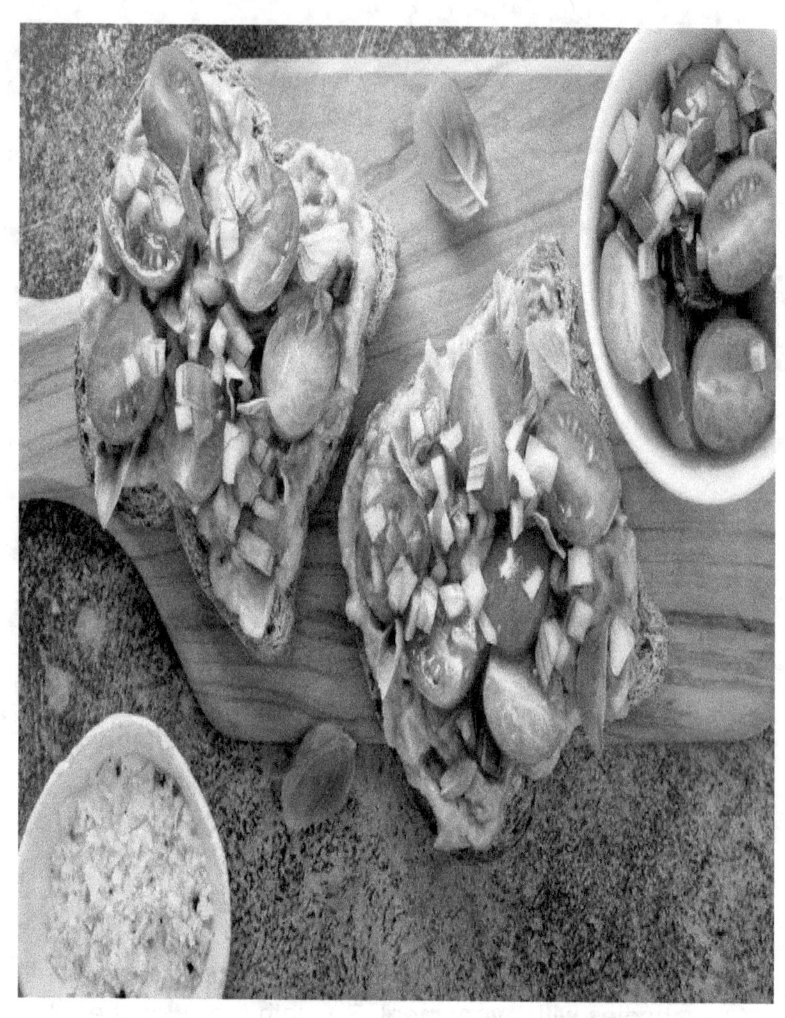

CHAPTER EIGHT

Snacks and Beverages for Liver Wellness

So far, still in our journey through the "Fatty Liver Diet Cookbook," we will be venturing into the delightful realm of snacks and beverages specially crafted to support liver wellness. From midday munchies to evening cravings, this chapter is your go-to guide for satisfying your appetite while nourishing your liver.

Welcome to a world where snacking isn't just about indulgence—it's about nourishment and care for your liver. In this chapter, we'll explore the importance of choosing snacks and beverages that promote liver health, providing you with energy, vitality, and a satisfying taste experience.

Understanding Liver-Friendly Snacks and Beverages

Before we embark on our culinary adventure, let's take a moment to understand what makes a snack or beverage liver-friendly. We'll explore the role of nutrients like antioxidants, fibre, and healthy fats in supporting liver function, as well as the importance of hydration in maintaining overall wellness. Armed with this knowledge, you'll be better equipped to make informed choices that benefit both your taste buds and your liver.

Recipes for Nourishment and Delight:
Now, let's get into the heart of the matter—the recipes! From crunchy snacks to refreshing beverages, we've curated a collection of options to suit every craving and dietary preference. Whether you're in the mood for a savoury treat, a sweet indulgence, or something in between, you'll find plenty of inspiration to satisfy your hunger and support your liver health.

Sample Recipes:

1. **Crunchy Chickpea Snack Mix:** Roasted chickpeas seasoned with a blend of herbs and spices make for a satisfyingly crunchy snack that's packed with protein and fibre. Enjoy this guilt-free treat on its own or as a topping for salads and soups.

2. **Berry Green Smoothie:** Start your day on the right foot with a refreshing green smoothie packed with antioxidant-rich berries, leafy greens, and a splash of coconut water. This vibrant beverage not only quenches your thirst but also provides a nourishing boost to your liver health.

3. **Avocado Toast with Tomato and Basil:** Elevate your snack game with a classic

avocado toast topped with juicy tomato slices and fresh basil. Rich in healthy fats, fibre, and vitamins, this simple yet satisfying snack is sure to become a staple in your repertoire.

Conclusion:

As you explore the world of snacks and beverages for liver wellness, remember that nourishment and enjoyment go hand in hand. With the recipes and insights shared in this chapter, you have the tools to make snack time a delicious and supportive part of your journey towards optimal liver health. So, indulge your cravings, sip on refreshing beverages, and savour every moment of nourishment and delight. Your liver—and your taste buds—will thank you for it.

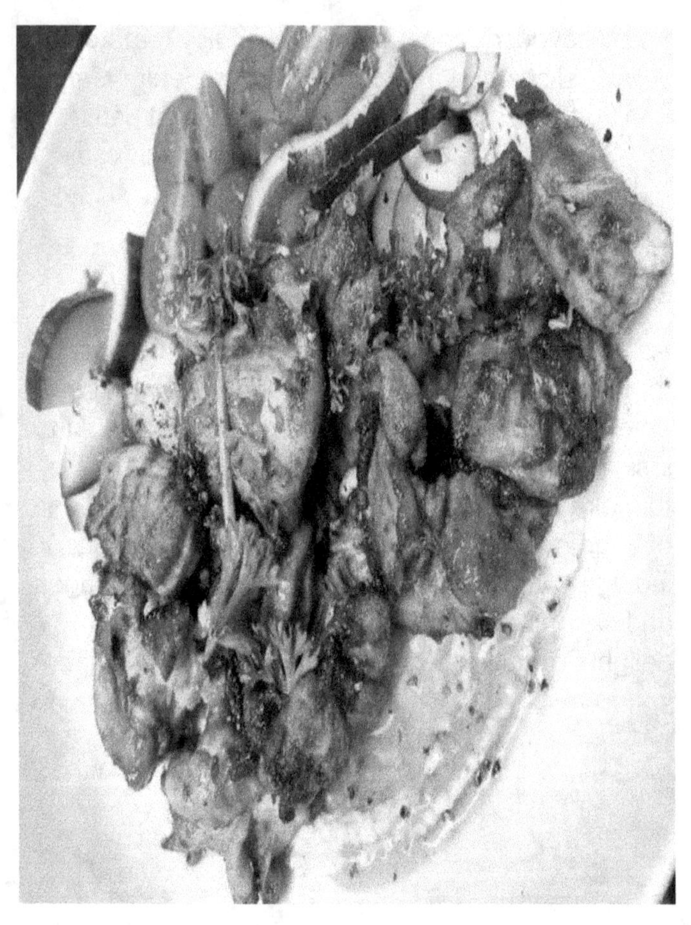

CHAPTER NINE

Desserts and Treats That Won't Harm Your Liver

Welcome to "Fatty Liver Diet Cookbook," where we're indulging our sweet tooth with desserts and treats that prioritise both flavour and liver health. In this chapter, we'll explore a world of decadent delights and guilt-free indulgences, proving that you can satisfy your cravings without compromising your liver wellness.

Desserts and treats often get a bad rap when it comes to liver health, but in reality, there's a wide array of options that can be enjoyed in moderation while still supporting your liver. In this chapter, we'll debunk the myth that healthy eating means saying goodbye to sweets, and instead, we'll show you how to indulge mindfully with recipes that nourish your body and tantalise your taste buds.

Finding Balance in Sweetness

Before we delve into the recipes, let's take a moment to discuss the importance of finding balance when it comes to desserts and treats. While it's true that excess sugar can be detrimental to liver health, enjoying occasional indulgences in moderation can be part of a balanced lifestyle. By choosing recipes that use wholesome ingredients and prioritise nutrient density, you can satisfy your sweet cravings while still supporting your liver wellness.

Recipes for Guilt-Free Indulgence

Now, let's get to the good stuff—the recipes! From decadent chocolate treats to fruity delights, we've curated a collection of desserts and treats that are as delicious as they are liver-friendly. Whether you're craving something rich and creamy or light and refreshing, you'll find plenty of options to satisfy your sweet tooth without harming your liver.

Sample Recipes

1. **Dark Chocolate Avocado Mousse:** Indulge your chocolate cravings with this creamy and decadent mousse made with ripe avocados, dark cocoa powder, and a touch of maple syrup. Rich in heart-healthy fats and antioxidants, this luscious dessert is a guilt-free way to satisfy your sweet tooth.

2. **Berry Yoghurt Parfait:** Layer tangy Greek yoghurt with fresh berries and a sprinkle of granola for a delightful parfait that's as nutritious as it is delicious. Packed with protein, fibre, and antioxidants, this dessert

is a refreshing treat that won't weigh you down.

3. **Frozen Banana Pops:** Dip banana slices in melted dark chocolate, sprinkle with chopped nuts or coconut flakes, and freeze for a satisfying frozen treat that's perfect for hot summer days. With the natural sweetness of bananas and the antioxidant power of dark chocolate, these popsicles are a wholesome indulgence you can feel good about.

Conclusion

As you explore the world of desserts and treats that won't harm your liver, remember that moderation is key. By choosing recipes that prioritise wholesome ingredients and mindful indulgence, you can enjoy sweet treats without compromising your liver health. So, whip up a batch of your favourite dessert, savour every bite, and celebrate the joy of nourishing your body while satisfying your sweet cravings. Your liver—and your taste buds—will thank you for it.

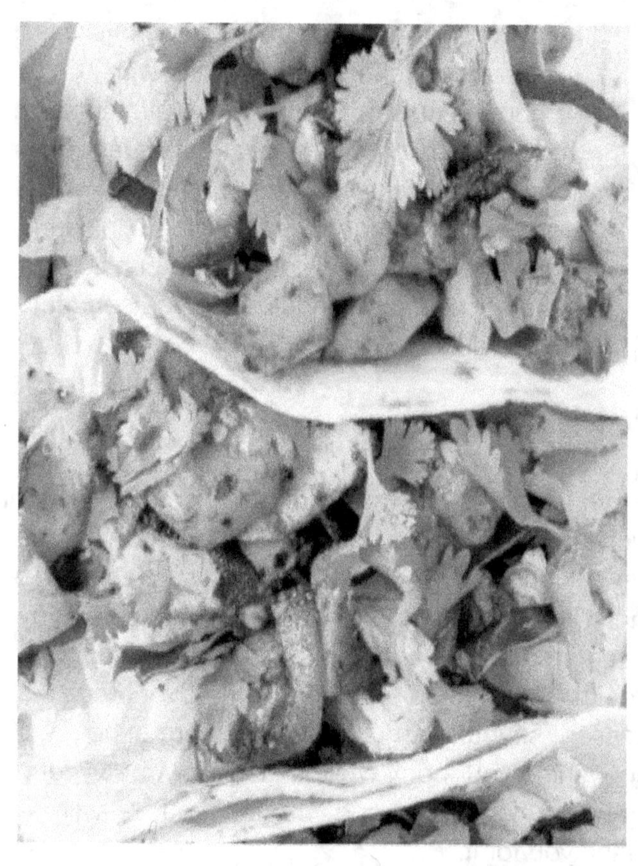

CHAPTER TEN

Meal Planning and Long-Term Maintenance for Fatty Liver Health

In this Chapter, we will embark on a journey of meal planning and long-term maintenance strategies to support liver health and overall well-being. As we have learned throughout this culinary adventure, nourishing our bodies and caring for our livers is not just about what we eat—it's about how we approach food, mealtime, and lifestyle choices. In this chapter, we'll delve into the art of meal planning, explore strategies for sustainable dietary habits, and discuss the importance of long-term maintenance in managing fatty liver health.

Meal planning is often seen as a daunting task, but in reality, it's a powerful tool for supporting liver health and promoting overall wellness. By taking the time to plan and prepare nourishing meals, we can ensure that we are fueling our bodies with the nutrients they need to thrive while minimising the risk of exacerbating fatty liver disease. In this chapter, we will explore the benefits of meal planning, provide practical tips for getting started, and discuss how to maintain healthy eating habits for the long term.

Before we delve into the nitty-gritty of meal planning, let's take a moment to discuss why it's so important for liver health. Fatty liver disease is often linked to poor dietary choices, including excessive consumption of processed foods, sugars, and unhealthy fats. By taking a proactive approach to meal planning, we can ensure that we're making thoughtful choices that support liver function and promote overall wellness. From balancing macronutrients to incorporating a variety of colourful fruits and vegetables, meal planning allows us to create a well-rounded diet that nourishes our bodies from within.

Getting Started with Meal Planning

Now that we understand the importance of meal planning, let's discuss how to get started. The key to successful meal planning is consistency, organisation, and flexibility. Begin by setting aside time each week to plan your meals, taking into account your schedule, dietary preferences, and nutritional needs. Make a list of recipes you'd like to try, create a shopping list, and batch cook ingredients to streamline meal preparation throughout the week. By investing a little time upfront, you will save yourself stress and ensure that you always have nutritious meals at the ready.

Meal planning is just one piece of the puzzle when it comes to maintaining a healthy lifestyle. To truly support liver health and promote long-term wellness, it's essential to cultivate sustainable dietary habits that can be maintained over time. This means focusing on whole, unprocessed foods, minimising the consumption of sugary beverages and snacks, and listening to your body's hunger and fullness cues. It also means finding balance in your diet, allowing yourself to enjoy occasional indulgences while prioritising nutrient-dense meals that nourish your body and support your liver.

The Role of Long-Term Maintenance

Finally, let's discuss the importance of long-term maintenance in managing fatty liver health. While meal planning and dietary changes can have a significant impact on liver function in the short term, it's essential to maintain these habits over the long term to see lasting results. This means adopting a lifestyle that prioritises healthy eating, regular physical activity, stress management, and adequate sleep. By incorporating these habits into your daily routine, you can support your liver health and overall well-being for years to come.

Summary

As we reach the conclusion of Chapter 8, it's clear that meal planning and long-term maintenance are essential components of managing fatty liver health. By taking a proactive approach to meal planning, cultivating sustainable dietary habits, and prioritising long-term maintenance, we can support our liver function, promote overall wellness, and live our best lives. So, embrace the power of meal planning, commit to healthy eating habits, and celebrate the journey towards optimal liver health. Your liver—and your whole body—will thank you for it.

CONCLUSION

As we close the final chapter of the "Fatty Liver Diet Cookbook," it's impossible not to reflect on the journey we've taken together—a journey of exploration, discovery, and transformation. Throughout these pages, we've delved deep into the complexities of managing fatty liver disease, exploring the role of nutrition, lifestyle, and mindful choices in supporting liver health and overall well-being. From understanding the fundamentals of a liver-friendly diet to crafting delicious and nutritious meals, from embracing the power of meal planning to cultivating sustainable dietary habits, we've covered a vast landscape of knowledge and insight.

At the heart of it all lies a simple yet profound truth: food is medicine, and what we choose to put on our plates has the power to heal, nourish, and rejuvenate our bodies from within. By embracing a diet rich in whole, unprocessed foods, prioritising nutrient density, and minimising the consumption of sugars, unhealthy fats, and processed foods, we can support our liver health and promote overall wellness. But beyond the realm of nutrition lies a deeper understanding—that true wellness extends beyond the plate, encompassing every aspect of our lives.

Throughout this culinary journey, we've explored the importance of holistic health, recognizing that optimal liver function is not achieved through diet alone but through a combination of factors, including regular physical activity, stress management, adequate sleep, and mindful living. By taking a comprehensive approach to wellness, we can nourish our bodies, nurture our minds, and cultivate a sense of balance and harmony that resonates throughout our entire being.

But perhaps the most profound lesson we've learned is that wellness is not a destination but a journey—a journey of self-discovery, growth, and self-care. It's about tuning into our bodies, listening to their needs, and honouring the wisdom they impart. It's about finding joy in the simple pleasures of nourishing meals, the company of loved ones, and the beauty of the world around us. It's about embracing imperfection, celebrating progress, and cultivating resilience in the face of life's challenges.

As we bid farewell to the pages of this cookbook, let us carry forward the lessons we've learned, the insights we've gained, and the recipes we've discovered. Let us continue to nourish our bodies with wholesome foods, nurture our minds with positive thoughts, and cultivate a lifestyle that honours the precious gift of health. And let us remember that we are not alone on this journey—that we have the support of our loved ones, the guidance of healthcare professionals, and the wisdom of generations past to light our way.

In the end, the "Fatty Liver Diet Cookbook" is not just a collection of recipes—it's a testament to the power of food as medicine, the resilience of the human spirit, and the infinite potential for healing and transformation that resides within each of us. So, as you embark on your own journey towards optimal liver health and overall wellness, remember to savour the flavours of life, embrace the joy of nourishment, and celebrate the miracle of being alive. Your liver—and your whole being—will thank you for it.

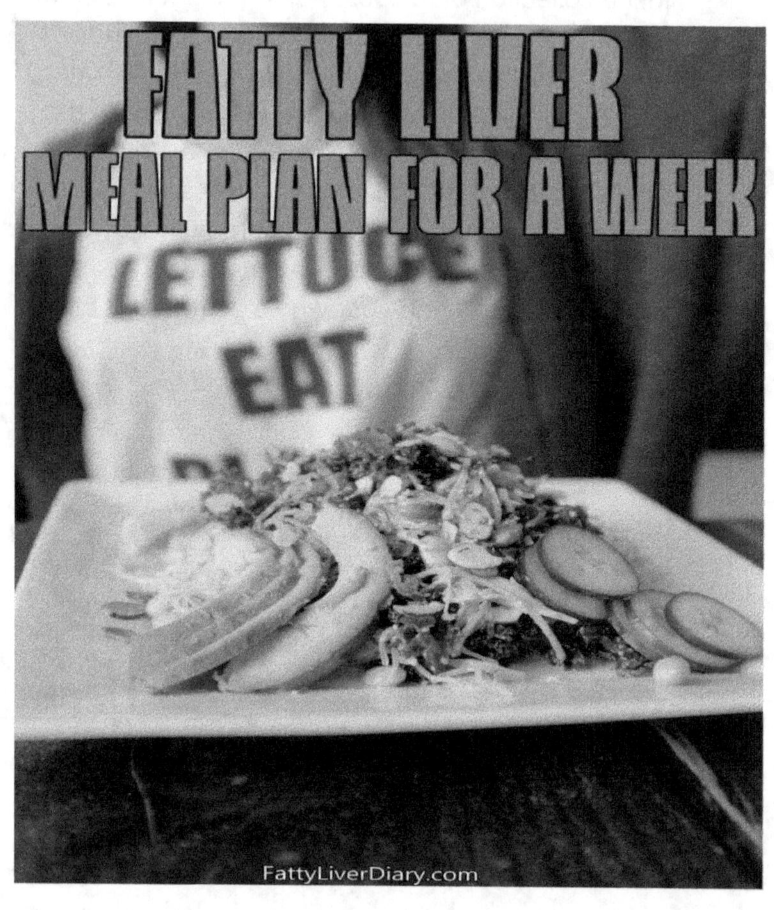

FATTY LIVER
MEAL PLAN FOR A WEEK
LETTUCE
EAT
FattyLiverDiary.com

www.ingramcontent.com/pod-product-compliance
Lightning Source LLC
Chambersburg PA
CBHW051848250726
48659CB00006B/2087